The Amazing Diet Secret of a Desperate Housewife

The Amazing Diet Secret of a Desperate Housewife

by
Nancy Pryor

A BRAND NEW REASON
TO LOSE WEIGHT

First of all, I want to say "thank you" for ordering this book. I believe that all too often people and companies who sell things forget or ignore common courtesy. And to me, a part of common courtesy says that you should let your customers know that you appreciate their business.

I *do* appreciate your business and I *am* grateful that you have placed enough faith in me to have ordered this book. Thanks again.

You are not going to be disappointed. Of course, I am prejudiced, but I believe this is about the best book you will ever find on the subject of losing weight. You are going to learn here some things you never knew before. Very important things.

You are going to learn how to lose weight fast and keep it off.

Not only that, I predict you will find it easier than you ever thought possible.

In addition to losing weight, you are going to learn about a healthier way of living that may add years to your life and life to your years.

You probably already have a lot of reasons for wanting to lose weight. Maybe you want to slim down so you will look and feel sexier and more attractive.

Maybe you are aware how unhealthy it is to be overweight and desire to get back to a good state of physical well being.

Maybe you want to lose weight just because you want to feel good about yourself.

Those are all good reasons and there are a lot more, but now I want to give you a brand new reason to lose weight.

The reason is money. Please let me explain:

As I very clearly state in my advertising, I am not a doctor, nor a nutritionist, nor anything like that. I am an ordinary garden variety housewife. But in spite of all that, I sincerely believe I have come up with a weight loss plan that outshines all the others.

But since I am *not* a doctor or anything, I need some help to prove how good my system is.

What I would like is for a lot of people to use my plan and then write me and tell me about the results.

I am going to pick out certain of those "success stories" and use them in my advertising.

And, of course, I will be happy to pay good money to anyone whose story I use in my advertising.

I figure I need about 50 success stories.

I want to use people who have lost a lot of weight *and* people who only needed to lose a few pounds.

3

I want to use both men and women. I'd like to have some older folks, some younger ones and some in between.

In other words, I want "success stories" from a good cross-section of people so that I can prove that my diet plan will work for just about anybody.

I want to know more than how much weight people have lost. I also want to know if their health has improved. I want to know if they feel better. Are they generally in a better mood? Are they less nervous? Do they have more energy? And so on.

Anyway, on the next few pages I have included a couple of forms that I hope you will fill out. These will help you keep track of your progress and also to organize your thinking if you want to write your own success story later on. There are two forms for women and two for men. You fill out the *before* form when you start the diet plan and the *after* form after you have lost the weight you wanted to lose. Here they are.

By the way, I'll be paying 50 dollars for some of the

4

success stories, $100 for others, $500 for others, and **$1,000** for the one I consider the best of all!

Before and After

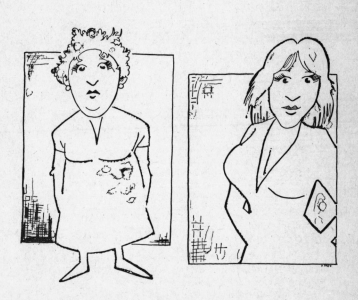

WOMEN
(BEFORE)

Age _____   Date _____

Height _____   + Morning Weight _____

Bust _____   Waist _____

Hips _____

How is your health in general? _____

What kind of a mood are you in most of the time?
Nervous? Depressed? Happy? Etc. _____

ENERGY: Do you usually feel peppy and
energetic? Or are you often draggy and lethargic?

_____

Dress Size _____ Signature _____

Note: It wouldn't hurt to take a picture of yourself
now so that after you have lost weight you'll
remember how you used to look.

+ Weigh yourself right after you get up after using
the bathroom and before you get dressed.

WOMEN
(AFTER)

Age _____   Date _____

Height _____   +Morning Weight _____

Bust _____   Waist _____

Hips _____

How is your health in general? _____

What kind of a mood are you in most of the time?
Nervous? Depressed? Happy? Etc. _____

ENERGY: Do you usually feel peppy and
energetic? Or are you often draggy and lethargic?
_____

Dress Size _____ Signature _____

Note: Why not take another picture of yourself now
so that you can compare it to how you used to look.

+ Weigh yourself right after you get up after using
the bathroom and before you get dressed.

7

MEN
(BEFORE)

Age _____   Date _____

Height _____   + Morning Weight _____

Chest _____   Waist _____

Hips _____

How is your health in general? _____

What kind of a mood are you in most of the time?
Nervous? Depressed? Happy? Etc. _____

ENERGY: Do you usually feel peppy and energetic?
Or are you often draggy and lethargic? _____

Signature _____

Note: It wouldn't hurt to take a picture of yourself
now so that after you have lost weight you'll
remember how you used to look.

+ Weigh yourself right after you get up and after
using the bathroom and before you get dressed.

8

MEN
(AFTER)

Age _____   Date _____

Height _____   + Morning Weight _____

Chest _____   Waist _____

Hips _____

How is your health in general? _____

What kind of a mood are you in most of the time?
Nervous? Depressed? Happy? Etc. _____

ENERGY: Do you usually feel peppy and energetic?
Or are you often draggy and lethargic? _____

Signature _____

Note: Why not take another picture of yourself now
so that you can compare it to how you used to look.

+ Weigh yourself right after you get up and after
   using the bathroom and before you get dressed.

9

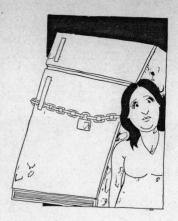

Deprivation Buildup

WHY IT'S SO HARD

Losing weight and keeping it off is very hard. In fact, for most people it seems to be impossible. Almost 100% of the people who go on a diet and lose weight eventually regain every pound and more than they have lost.

It is much harder to lose weight and keep it off than it is to give up smoking, or stop drinking, or even to overcome most drug addictions.

Here's why.

Let's say you are a heavy smoker and you want to give up cigarettes. There is no doubt it will be hard. As the nicotine in your body is flushed out, you will suffer very real and unpleasant withdrawal symptoms. The first few days will be brutal. You will crave a cigarette with every cell in your body. But if you can hold out for a week, your desire for a cigarette will be less and less each day. After about three weeks when nearly all of the residual nicotine has left your body, you will only crave a cigarette a couple of times a day. And even then, the craving will become less and less intense. As time goes on, you will suddenly notice that you haven't even thought about smoking for days on end. And then weeks on end.

In other words, when you give up smoking, every day it gets easier. The same is true of alcohol and drugs.

With dieting it's just the opposite. *Every day it gets harder!*

Here's why.

Let's say you need to lose 25 pounds and by God, this time you've made up your mind to do it. You pick out a nice healthy 1,000 calorie a day diet and you resolve to stay on it no matter what.

The first day is not so bad. You are excited about your new diet and the idea of looking slim and trim again.

The next few days aren't so bad either. Sure you get hungry every so often, and you are never quite satisfied, but you can handle it.

After all, it's worth a little sacrifice to start looking and feeling good again. Right?

However, after about a week, the newness of the diet has worn off. You are no longer so excited and enthusiastic. You *are*, however, still hungry a lot. In fact, you are feeling hungrier and more and more deprived every day.

But you are strong. You hang in there.

But sooner or later, after X number of days or X number of weeks of constant gnawing hunger and of feeling deprived all the time, you give in.

One day you say to yourself, "to hell with it". I'm going to have at least one satisfying meal. Maybe one piece of cake or a dish of ice cream.

And so you do. And then you feel guilty. And then you get on the scale. And then you feel even more guilty because you have regained so much in so little time.

And then because you feel so bad, you eat more.

And soon you are right back where you started. Eventually, if you are like most people, after a while you will be ashamed once again to be so fat and you will look around for yet another diet and start all over.

Unfortunately, you will probably get the same results.

You see, my friend, you are fighting a losing battle. You are trying to defeat constant hunger and what I call "deprivation buildup" with will power.

It can't be done.

And even if you could - so what? What good is it to

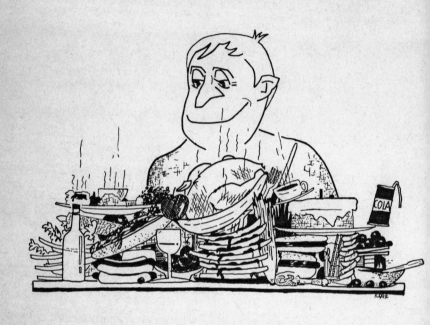

be trim and slim if you are miserable and hungry all the time? What kind of a life is that?

What you really need is a diet strategy that sees to it that you are *never* hungry. Also, you need a plan that lets you get some fun out of life. As every dieter knows, when you are hungry for a piece of cake or ice cream or a baked potato with butter, then that is *exactly* what you *must* have in order to feel satisfied. Lettuce and carrots just won't get the job done.

If you don't get what you want, you will feel deprived. It's just that simple. And you *cannot* diet successfully if you go around feeling hungry and/or deprived all the time.

Is there such a plan? Is there a weight loss system that makes sure you are *never* hungry? One that lets you eat your cake and lose weight too?

Yes there is. In a few pages I will reveal it to you. But first it is *very important* that you understand a few things about eating and dieting and body chemistry that no one ever told you before. It is especially important that you understand hunger, so let's start with that.

WHY YOU GET HUNGRY

You get hungry when your blood sugar is low. It's not so much how full your stomach is that makes you hungry. It's how full your bloodstream is - with sugar. If you have low blood sugar, you will not only be hungry, you will also very likely be tense and irritable. Naturally, you will be low on energy.

All of this causes you to crave food. And, of course, the way to elevate your blood sugar is to eat. And the fastest way, of course, is to eat something that contains sugar, or starch that is quickly converted to sugar. In other words, the best way to get rid of hunger is to eat some candy or cake or ice cream or bread and butter or potatoes and gravy, and so on.

There's a big problem with this, however. And it's not what you think. It's *not* so much the calories. But rather it's the reaction your body has to sugar. You see, sugar is relatively low in calories. It has only 16 per

16

teaspoonful, but sugar often starts a dangerous and unhealthy chain reaction in your body.

Here's how it works:

Your blood sugar is low and you are hungry. You are at a movie so you eat a couple of candy bars. Soon you are content. The sugar from the candy enters your bloodstream quite rapidly and you are no longer hungry, tense and irritable.

So far so good.

However, very soon all this sugar in your bloodstream causes your body to produce insulin. Insulin is used by the body to regulate the level of sugar in your blood. So, if your blood sugar is *too* high, your body will produce insulin that pulls the excess sugar out of your bloodstream and stores it in your liver for later use.

This is all fine and dandy for people who are more or less "biochemically normal."

But many, perhaps most, overweight people are not "biochemically normal." When *their* blood sugar is high, many overweight people produce *too much insulin too fast*! And this causes, not only the *excess* sugar, but nearly all of the energy giving sugar to be removed from the blood.

Guess what happens then?

You are right. Since nearly *all* the sugar is pulled out of the bloodstream, you are hungry all over again. And low on energy. And irritable. And tense.

Perhaps even more so than you were before you ate the candy bars.

And what's the best way to appease that hunger and increase your energy and get rid of that tenseness and irritability?

Right again. Eat some sugary or starchy food.

And then, of course, it starts all over again - a vicious cycle that keeps you eating almost constantly.

So the first thing you must do if you are to diet successfully is to raise your blood sugar level so that you will not be hungry. But, that alone is not enough. You must also do this in a way that will not induce an insulin response which will take most of the sugar right back out of your bloodstream.

And that brings us to the first big secret of my weight loss system. Here it is in one word:

SECRET #1

FRUCTOSE

Fructose is fruit sugar. It is a remarkable food substance. It looks and tastes exactly like ordinary table sugar (sucrose). At least it does to me. Some people say it's a little sweeter than sucrose. Fructose has the same number of calories as sucrose. You can use it in exactly the same way you normally use your table sugar.

But when fructose enters your body, it has a very different affect on you than ordinary sugar.

First of all, fructose is more slowly absorbed into your bloodstream than ordinary sugar. Also, unlike other sugars, it can be assimilated *directly* into your muscle cells.

19

The most important thing for you to remember, however is that *fructose raises your blood sugar level without inducing an insulin response*!

Just think of what that means! It means that when you are hungry, you can eat or drink something sweet to raise your blood sugar level and get rid of the hunger. *And* if something sweet is fructose, not only will your blood sugar level go up, it will stay up.

In other words - now at last - you can eat something sweet to satisfy your hunger and your hunger will *stay* satisfied!

So the first thing we are going to do is to add fructose to your diet every day. I'll tell you exactly how and how much a little later on. I'll also tell you where to get fructose and how much it costs and how to use it, and so on.

But for now, be happy. You have just learned one of the major secrets of my weight loss system. Believe me, it is an important one. It means that from now on you can lose weight and keep it off without *ever* having to go hungry.

As I said, we'll talk more about exactly how to use fructose a little later on, but right now let's go on to the second big secret. Here it is in a nutshell:

SECRET #2
DON'T DIET EVERY DAY —
INSTEAD, DIET EVERY OTHER DAY!

Sounds simple, doesn't it? It is. But it is also a very important concept. Please let me explain.

Normally, when you go on a diet, you do so with the idea of staying on the diet *every day* until you are down to your proper weight. This sounds good in theory but in practice it is almost impossible.

It is almost impossible because of what I call "deprivation buildup."

"Deprivation buildup" is what happens when you eat less than you want every day for days on end.

I mentioned earlier how every day that you stay on a "normal" low calorie diet, you get hungrier and

21

hungrier. You start feeling more and more deprived. Sooner or later you give in and then - WHAM - you start binge eating to make up for all that suffering.

But imagine what it would be like if you only had to diet every other day.

First of all, contrary to popular opinion, overweight people often have *more* willpower than slim people. It would be a snap for most overweight people to go on an extremely strict diet if they only had to stay on it for one day. After all, most overweight people have gone on one or another starvation diet for days, or weeks before they finally gave in.

But with the every other day idea, you only have to "suffer" one day at a time. Would you not agree that it would be much easier to go on a strict diet Monday if you knew you could eat pretty much anything you wanted all day Tuesday?

Of course it would. And not only that - as soon as you learn how to use fructose, you won't even have to "suffer" on your diet day!

Like I said, this is a very simple idea. But once again let me stress that it is a very important idea. You see, this way you can diet Monday, eat normally Tuesday - and then diet again Wednesday without any "deprivation buildup" at all. You could actually keep going like this forever. You've got to admit it would be a lot easier this way than to try to stay on any diet for weeks on end without ever giving yourself a break.

Actually, this one single idea can make it possible for you to stay on *any* diet for as long as you like.

You really don't need to read any more of this book to start losing weight very effectively. You could be successful if you would only use the information I have given you so far. After all, it is easy to stay on almost any diet if you only have to do it every other day - especially if you can use fructose whenever you start to get hungry.

But I want to make it even easier and more enjoyable for you so let's move right on to secret number three. By the way, in a few more pages I am going to lay out everything for you in an easy step-by-step plan. I will tell you *exactly* what to do. But in the meantime, please bear with me because I want you to *understand* the principles involved. OK, now let's move along. Here is secret number three:

SECRET #3

NATURAL FOOD TRANQUILIZERS

Fructose, by itself, seems to be very soothing to the nerves. However, there are certain other foods and food substances that also have a tranquilizing affect on the body. I call these foods "natural food tranquilizers" but that probably is not scientifically correct.

But what is correct for sure is that these foods are very good for you. They give you uncommon energy, they make you feel better and they have a calming affect that makes it much easier to diet and to live with stress in general.

Incidentally, dieting does cause stress, no matter what the makeup of the diet. That is because a new diet is a change and any change causes stress. It doesn't matter if the change is good or bad. It causes stress either way.

Most everyone gets irritable and out of sorts when they try to diet. This is one of the major reasons people go off their diets. In this section I am going to tell you about some things that can help you with this problem. Then later on I will put it all together and tell you exactly how to add them to your diet.

LECITHIN

There are at least two important reasons to include lecithin in your diet plans. One reason is lecithin's marvelous tranquilizing effect and the other is lecithin's ability to redistribute weight from where it's unwanted to where it's needed.

Lecithin is pronounced "less-i-thin." it is a concentrated nerve nutrient extracted from soybeans. It comes in the form of a granular powder. It can be sprinkled on food or mixed in liquids. It also comes in capsules. It is an extremely important factor in the digestion and oxidation of fats.

Many of the nerve fibers in your body are surrounded by a protective cover called the myelin sheath. This sheath is rich in lecithin. If you don't get enough lecithin, your nerves will not be properly cushioned and protected and they will become irritated.

On the other hand, if you supply your body with a generous supply of lecithin everyday, your nerves will be soothed and you may very likely discover yourself to be a much calmer person.

That's not all. Doctors maintain that lecithin does a lot more. They say it nourishes your nerve cells, combats fatigue, irritability and brain fag, and can even reverse cases of sexual decline and nervous exhaustion. They say it produces more alertness, lowers blood pressure, softens aging skin and keeps your skin in good shape while reducing.

It is a *crucial* food substance for people who are prone to heart attacks as it is nature's number one cholesterol emulsifier.

You see, lecithin helps prevent hardening of the arteries by loosening up the gobules of fat so they can move on and be flushed out of your body instead of settling on your artery walls.

Lecithin is *not* a synthetic chemical product. It is a lifesaving substance and a potent tranquilizing brain food.

DOLOMITE

Dolomite is a combination of the minerals calcium and magnesium. It is prepared from a special natural limestone which is mined deep in the earth to prevent contamination. It is available in tablet form.

Calcium and magnesium are magnificent mineral relaxers of jangled nerves. In fact, one of the major causes of nervousness in all ages is a calcium deficiency.

Most of the calcium (99%) in your body is in your bones and teeth. But the 1% that is needed by your nervous system can make life unbearable if it isn't there.

The blood of people who suffer from extreme irritability has been found to be low in calcium.

Calcium is an excellent pain killer and can help greatly in overcoming grouchiness and insomnia.

Some people call calcium tablets their "natural lullaby pills."

In general, calcium aids in the smooth transmission of nerve impulses and will contribute a lot to your all around peace of mind.

Magnesium is a mineral of many resources. It also helps relax the nerves and smooths nerve impulse transmission and helps control blood cholesterol. In addition, it influences the metabolism of calcium. Believe me, these two important minerals combined in dolomite pills are going to make a big difference in your diet.

POWDERED BREWERS YEAST

Powdered brewers yeast is the dried pulverized cells of the yeast plant. it is a complete food and the finest source of B vitamins found in nature. It is nearly all protein. It contains no sugar and no fat and almost no starch. Ounce for ounce, it is probably the most nutritious food in the world for human consumption.

The B vitamins in yeast are complete and in the correct natural proportions. Powdered yeast is a much better source of B vitamins than B vitamin pills.

Stress uses up the B vitamins in your body, so consequently, powdered yeast is perhaps the very best food you can eat in times of stress.

And as I intend to keep pointing out to you, dieting *is* a stress, under even the best of conditions. No matter what diet you go on, it will be a change, and therefore a stress.

It is impossible to be at peace with yourself when you are feeling a lot of stress, and that is why I am emphasizing these "natural food tranquilizers" in this section.

I also want to point out that not only will these foods make you feel better, they are also very good for you.

A heaping tablespoonful of yeast contains 20 grams of perfect complete protein. In addition to soothing your nerves, it will work to satisfy your appetite, provide energy, and to regulate your basal metabolism.

Do not take uncooked baker's yeast by mistake as a substitute for powdered brewers yeast. They are not the same. And uncooked baker's yeast is not good for you.

By the way, when you first start adding yeast to your diet, you may find it hard to digest and you may get a little gas. If so, this is a sign that you are in desperate need of yeast and the B vitamins it provides.

I'll explain exactly how to add yeast to your diet just a little later on. But first, let's go on to the other food substances.

YOGURT

Nearly everybody is familiar with yogurt and almost everyone has some idea that it is very good for you. Many more people eat it regularly now that frozen yogurt parlors have become so popular.

This is a healthy trend because yogurt is very good for you. Even the frozen kind that contains sugar is better for you than ice cream.

Yogurt is a predigested custard-like milk product. It contains lacto-bacillus bacteria which destroys putrefactive bacteria and it is a distinct aid to proper digestion. Because of this, it is an especially excellent food for people who have bad breath and are prone to gas.

Yogurt is good for you in many ways. It is an excellent source of perfect complete protein. It has all the vitamins and minerals of milk in a much more easily digested form than regular milk.

But the main reason I am writing about it here is because it is another of those wonderful "natural food tranquilizers."

Each 8 ounces contains 250 milligrams of already dissolved calcium and we have already discussed how important calcium is to your nerves. But to me, the best thing about yogurt is how it helps you to digest all the other foods and vitamins and nutrients you take into your system.

You know, it's not the nutrients that you eat that makes you healthy - it's the nutrients you digest.

It doesn't matter if you eat good food if you can't digest it properly. That's one of the reasons so many Americans are "overfed and undernourished."

Since yogurt helps you digest and absorb the nutrients you eat and because it has so many good things itself (including all that soothing calcium), it very much deserves to be included in this section on "natural food tranquilizers."

WHEAT GERM

Scientists have not yet caught up with nature. I suspect they never will. As a result, no one really knows exactly everything that a person needs for perfect nutrition.

We can take a particular food and scientifically examine it and identify many of its individual nutrients. But you know, there are many important trace elements in a lot of foods that we *cannot* identify.

One of the sorriest things we ever learned how to do is to make white flour. When we make white flour, we mostly refine out all the good stuff. The main thing we refine out is the wheat embryo or wheat germ. It is this germ of the wheat that contains nearly all of the nutrition of wheat.

We can, of course, add synthetic vitamins to the flour and then say it is "enriched." But it is never really the same nor as good as the original real thing that nature put together for us in the first place.

The germ of the wheat contains a lot of B vitamins and a lot of vitamin E. I strongly suspect it also contains a lot of other unidentified anti-stress factors.

For this reason, I would like for you to add it to your diet program.

Not only is it good for you - it is good tasting.

It can be added to your diet in many ways. I like to eat it as a cereal sweetened with fructose.

I have specific recommendations of exactly how and how much to add to your diet and just a little later on we'll get to them in the section I keep promising you where we are going to put all this together.

SECRET #4

EAT BEFORE YOU EAT

This is another of those ideas that is so simple and so good that you'll wonder why you didn't come up with it yourself.

As we have already seen, it is low blood sugar that makes you hungry. It takes about 20 minutes for your blood sugar to rise after you start to eat.

This means that if you eat enough to satisfy your hunger in the first five minutes of a meal, that you won't know it for another 15 minutes. As a result, you will continue to eat and most likely overeat during those remaining 15 minutes.

The way to get around this is to eat before you eat. If you intend to eat supper at 7:30, you should prepare yourself by pre-eating something at 7 o'clock.

That way when you sit down to eat, your blood sugar will have already started to rise. As a result, you will be much less likely to overeat.

What this technique does, in effect, is to more or less put you in touch with your *real* food needs. It also calms you down and helps to take the hysteria out of eating.

With the use of fructose, this idea becomes even more effective.

Once again, I'll tell you exactly how to use this idea in a few more pages. In the meantime, let's go on to the next secret.

SECRET #5

KELP

Adele Davis, the world famous nutritionist, has written that all sick people, all people with high blood cholesterol, *and all overweight people* need extra iodine.

Kelp is the best source of organic iodine. It is a natural salt substitute made from certain seaweeds. In addition to iodine, it also contains calcium, potassium and various trace minerals.

If you do not get enough iodine, your thyroid gland will not function properly and it is your thyroid gland that determines the speed at which your energy is produced. If your thyroid gland is sluggish, your metabolism (body energy) will be low and you won't burn up the food you eat as fast as you would otherwise.

Adding just one teaspoon of granular kelp to your diet each day will help to insure that your thyroid gland has all the iodine it needs to function properly.

This is very important to everyone who is trying to lose weight. Nothing is more frustrating than eating very little and still not losing weight simply because you have a slow metabolism.

That concludes the section on natural food tranquilizers. Now that you have a better idea of the secrets or "tools" we are going to use to help you lose weight, we are ready to move on to the specific diet plans.

There are three of these plans. Plan #1 is the fastest. Plan #2 is a little slower but more appealing to some people. Plan #3 actually lets you develop your own diet according to certain guidelines.

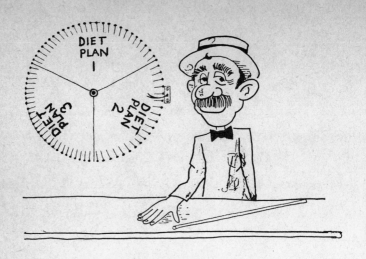

PLAN #1

THE FASTEST

This is the fastest of the three diet plans I am going to reveal to you. As with all of the plans, you only diet every other day. However, there are certain guidelines you must follow even on the so-called "eating days." I'll explain those guidelines in a moment.

But let's take the "diet days" first. On this plan, every diet day is the same and they are very simple. All you have is six glasses of fruit juice. And that's it. Nothing else. No solid food at all.

38

If you wish, you may sweeten each glass of juice with two teaspoons of fructose. You may choose from any of the following juices: apple, orange, papaya, pear, mango, or peach.

Try to get fresh juice. If you must use canned juice, be very sure that no sugar or artificial sweeteners have been added. Use only one kind of juice all day. You can switch juices if you like each new diet day, but only use one kind on any given day.

In addition to the fruit juices, you may have other beverages such as tea, coffee and diet colas so long as they do not contain any calories.

You can have these beverages if you like, but I hope you don't.

Here's why.

You probably want to lose weight so you will look better. But, you know, there is more to looking good than being slim. If you have nothing but fruit juices every other day, you will be giving your body a long needed break. You see fruit juice requires almost no digestion and therefore, your body will be able to use this time to do some "housecleaning." It will have a chance to digest and flush out some of the unnatural chemicals and mildly toxic poisons your body has been accumulating for such a long time. This will make you look and feel a lot better. Your skin will especially benefit. It will clear up, soften, and look much younger.

If you drink coffee, tea, and diet beverages, it will not slow down your weight loss, but it *will* add more unneeded chemicals to your system. It is also amazing how much better you will look if you stop taking in these substances.

However, like I said, you'll lose weight either way so it's up to you.

Now let's talk about your "eating days." On your eating days, I'm going to tell you exactly what to have for breakfast, and lunch. At supper you can pretty much eat the same way you do right now. I'm not going to take any of your favorite foods away from you during this meal, but I will ask, however, that you don't start eating *more* than you do right now.

In addition, I'm going to ask that you follow certain rules about your diet. This is very important.

First of all, I want you to have one level tablespoonful of fructose 20 minutes before each of your meals. You can have it in coffee, tea, fruit juice, or, if you wish, simply mixed in water. My favorite way to take fructose is to mix it with a glass of water and the juice of half a lemon. This "fructose lemonade" is sweet and delicious.

Anyway, however you take the fructose - TAKE IT! This is an ironclad rule. Then, 15 minutes later, when you sit down to eat, get in the habit of paying attention to yourself. When you notice during the meal that you **are truly no longer hungry - try and stop eating.**

In addition to your "fructose cocktail," I want you to substitute a health milk shake for your regular breakfast. This milk shake is made primarily of the ingredients I listed in the section on natural food tranquilizers. Here's how you make it.

Put 1½ glasses of skim milk into a blender. Then add:

1 tablespoon safflower oil (this will flush out excess water from your body)

1 tablespoon fructose

1 teaspoon vanilla extract

Then start the blender on low and add:

1 tablespoon powdered yeast

1 tablespoon lecithin

You can mix this up and drink it immediately. However, it will taste better if you mix it up one day and put it in the refrigerator overnight and then drink it the next day after you whip it up again for about 30 seconds. The overnight cold seems to make the yeast taste better. In other words, the best idea is to whomp up this concoction on your diet day and actually drink it on your eating day.

This milk shake serves two purposes. First of all, it has a lot of good stuff in it that will not only improve your health, but also have a welcome relaxing effect on your nerves. The other thing is that it will help curb your appetite. The fructose, yeast and milk protein contained in this drink are three of the most potent hunger fighters known to man.

Okay, that's breakfast. For lunch, you get one serving (1 cup) of plain yogurt sweetened with 1 teaspoon of fructose and topped with one tablespoon of wheat germ. Also, you get one piece of fruit. I suggest you cut up the fruit and add it to the yogurt, but you may eat it separately if you prefer. By the way, make sure that the yogurt you buy is plain, *low fat,* yogurt.

That's lunch. Now for supper, as I've told you, you can eat pretty much the same way you do now. I'm not going to go back on that statement, but there are a few rules that you *must* follow.

Here they are:

1. Be sure to have your tablespoon of fructose 15 minutes before you eat.

2. Always include vegetables with your supper. I don't care if you have them in salad or if you have them cooked, but do have them.

3. Take one teaspoon of granular kelp with this meal. Don't worry - it doesn't taste bad at all. You can use it in place of salt to season your food.

4. Take 3 dolomite pills after you eat. Also, if you take vitamins (and I hope you do), now is the time to take them.

There are no snacks permitted on this plan and when you are finished with supper, you are finished eating for the day. Eat enough to satisfy yourself but try not to overeat.

This is a good plan to follow if you want a fast weight loss without taking chances with your health. In fact, it is a good diet plan *and* a good health building plan. Now, just to make sure everything is clear, I'm going to sum it all up for you in outline form.

DIET DAY

Drink six 8 ounce glasses of fruit juice. Use only one type of juice per day. Each glass may be sweetened with one or two teaspoons of fructose. You may have other beverages, such as black coffee, tea and diet colas so long as they contain no calories. Naturally, you may drink all the water you like. Don't eat or drink anything else and don't take any vitamins or supplements.

EATING DAY

Breakfast   Health Milk Shake

Lunch   Yogurt - 1 cup plain, low fat, sweetened with 1 teaspoon fructose, topped off with 1 tablespoon wheat germ.

Fruit - 1 piece eaten separately or cut up and added to yogurt.

Supper   Fructose - 1 tablespoon 15 minutes before eating, mixed with any no calorie beverage.

Granular Kelp - Use 1 teaspoon to season food.

Vegetables - In salads or cooked, but have some for sure.

Other Foods - Eat whatever you like but pay attention to yourself and try and stop eating when you are no longer hungry.

Dolomite - Take 3 pills right after eating.

Vitamins - Take right after eating.

Snacks   None - On this plan, when you are finished eating supper, you are finished eating for the day.

NOTES

This diet brings hunger to a full dead stop. You will never be hungry. As a matter of fact, one of the unique features of this diet makes it metabolically impossible for you to experience hunger. To me, it's like heaven. The six teaspoons of fructose added to your juice should be enough to keep you from getting hungry on your diet days. Of course, you can always have an additional teaspoon of fructose with a no calorie beverage whenever you feel like it.

This diet converts body fat into body fuel. My experience is that my energy seems to increase starting about the fifth day of the diet and then it continues to increase until about the ninth day when it begins to level off. I would guesstimate that my new level is about 70 to 80% higher than it was before the diet. Now, if you want an easier plan with a somewhat slower weight loss, go on to Plan #2.

PLAN #2

FAST, BUT NOT QUITE SO FAST

The eating day on this plan is exactly the same as the one in Plan #1. However, the diet day is different. Instead of juice, you will have three small meals and one snack. Here they are:

Breakfast	Eggs - Have 2 poached or boiled.
	Toast - 1 slice whole wheat lightly buttered.
	Fruit - 1 piece any type (use fresh fruit, not something out of a can with sugar added).
Lunch	Salad - 1 large green with Italian dressing.
	Yogurt - 1 pint plain sweetened with 1 teaspoon fructose and topped off with 1 tablespoon wheat germ.
Supper	Chicken or Fish - 6 ounces of either - baked or broiled.
	Granular Kelp - Use one teaspoon to season fish or chicken.
	Vegetables - Raw or steamed - anything but potatoes or beans.
	Bread - 1 slice whole wheat lightly buttered.
Snack	Popcorn - 2 cups lightly salted - no butter.

NOTES

Be sure to take one teaspoon of fructose with a no calorie beverage before each meal and whenever you *first start* to get hungry. On this plan, you take your vitamins and dolomite pills both on your eating day *and* your diet day.

PLAN #3

ROLL YOUR OWN

I am going to give you a list of seven rules. You can make up your own diet and lose weight quite rapidly so long as you follow these guidelines. Here are the rules:

1. **DIET ONLY EVERY OTHER DAY.**

    This is important. If you follow this rule, you can stay on just about any diet for as long as you wish. After all, anybody can hold out for one day if they know that as soon as they wake up, they can have pretty much whatever they want for breakfast.

51

2. HAVE ONE TEASPOON FRUCTOSE 15 MINUTES BEFORE EACH MEAL ON BOTH YOUR DIET DAYS AND YOUR EATING DAYS AND ALSO ANYTIME YOU FIRST START TO GET HUNGRY. Believe me, this is going to be more of a help than you now know.

3. DON'T EAT SUCROSE (TABLE SUGAR) OR ANYTHING MADE WITH SUCROSE. You don't have to now because you have fructose to take its place. *But fructose will not effectively curb your hunger if you eat ordinary sugar along with it.* The reason is that the sucrose will induce an insulin response even if the fructose does not. You are going to have to be careful about this rule because there is sugar hidden in almost everything. Check labels very carefully.

4. DON'T EAT ANYTHING THAT IS MADE WITH WHITE FLOWER.

White flower is very quickly converted to sugar (not fruit sugar) right after it enters your system. Therefore, it can cause an insulin response.

5. START ADDING ALL OF THE "NATURAL FOOD TRANQUILIZERS" TO YOUR DIET.

Dieting is hard enough as it is. Don't make it worse by letting yourself get tense. Not only will these foods help to soothe your nerves, they will also provide you with a lot of good nutrition.

6. **ADD ONE TEASPOON OF GRANULAR KELP TO YOUR DIET EVERY DAY.** Give yourself every break you can. Adding kelp to your diet will help make sure you have enough iodine to "burn off" the food you eat.

7. **PAY ATTENTION TO YOURSELF AND TRY TO STOP EATING WHEN YOU ARE NO LONGER HUNGRY.**
   This is especially important on your "eating days." Most dieters are secretly hysterical about eating. Try and remember that this isn't the last meal you are ever going to have. Remember also that from now on, you only have to diet one day at a time. Try and slow down.

That's it. If you follow these rules, you should be able to develop a diet that is tailor made for you. Not only that, by following the every other day plan, you should be able to stay on your diet as long as necessary without undue discomfort. The addition of the fructose and natural food tranquilizers should go a long way toward taking the edge off your hunger and also to help you achieve a nice peaceful easy feeling. This is a Godsend for dieters.

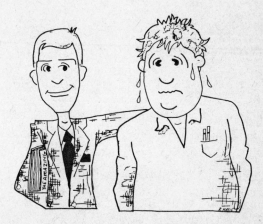

Boy, do I have something for you to read.

A FINAL WORD

Now you know all the "secrets" and you have all of the "tools" that you need in order to lose weight successfully. They have worked for me and I feel sure they will work for you. Some of these ideas are deceptively simple. But don't let that fool you. Often, the simplest ideas are the best.

The most important thing is to take care of your health. Everybody is different. Some foods are very good for one person and bad for another. So don't start on these or any other diet plans without checking first with your doctor. This is *your* responsibility. Nobody can do it for you.

Try to make your dieting as automatic as possible so that you don't have to think about it. This is especially easy with the every other day diet ideas.

All of the food substances mentioned in this book should be available at any good health food store. If you have trouble finding fructose, you can order it by mail from:

Valley Forge Health Products

4 B Progress Drive

Montgomeryville, Pa. 18936

They have it in both tablet and granular form. I suggest you write them for their current prices.

Well that's all I have to say, except "Good Luck!"

I really hope you are successful. My heart is with you. Believe me, I know how hard it is to diet. If you have any "secrets" you would like to share with me. or if you want to send in your "success story", you can write me. The address is:

Nancy Pryor

18 Lackawanna Plaza

Montclair, New Jersey 07042

I started this book by saying "thank you" and that's how I want to finish it. So "thanks" once again and may God be with you.

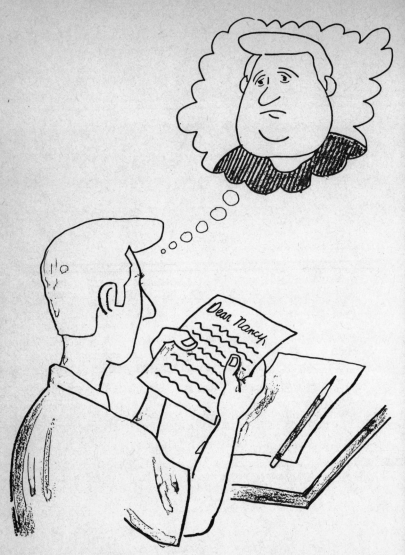

"Don't forget we'd like to hear from you."
—Nancy Pryor

WARNING!!!

The diet plans explained in this book have been carefully researched and they have been used by thousands of people without ill effects.

However, *every* diet plan and *every* food is dangerous for somebody.

Even staples such as milk, potatoes, orange juice and bread are contraindicated for certain people.

Therefore, you should check with your doctor before going on *any* new diet.

The information presented here is based upon the latest up-to-date scientific, diet, health, and nutritional information available. Even though the information presented here is based upon natural food substances, the author or publisher assumes no liability resulting from its application.

Always consult a doctor where matters of health are concerned.

This diet is no exception. It is especially important that you get your doctor's assurance that the fructose will not aggrevate any blood sugar abnormalities you may have such as hypoglycemia or diabetes.

Even though fructose does not produce an insulin response as does sugar and is much healthier for you than sugar, if you suffer from hypoglycemia or diabetes you may not be able to use fructose or any sugar substance as outlined in this diet.

Printed on the following pages are day by day "Cheat Sheets".

There is no need for you to fill out these sheets **unless** you go off your diet.

But if you ever do go off the diet, fill in the sheet for that day. This will help you to stop kidding yourself about how much you overeat.

I suggest that every day you stay on the diet, you give yourself a little reward by making a big fat X where it says "Good for me! Once again I stayed on my diet!".

Somehow it is very satisfying to make that big X at the end of every successful day. At least it is for me.

Of course, you may want to use the sheets as sort of a diet diary and record your daily moods, thoughts and ideas in the remarks section.

If so, that's fine, but whatever you do, be **sure** to fill out the sheet **anytime** you cheat.

It is very important that you be honest with yourself.

CHEAT SHEET

☐ Good for me! Once again I stayed on my diet!

☐ I cheated. Here is a list of what I ate or drank that wasn't on my diet.

_____   _____

_____   _____

_____   _____

_____   _____

_____   _____

Remarks: _____

_____

_____

_____

CHEAT SHEET

☐ Good for me! Once again I stayed on my diet!

☐ I cheated. Here is a list of what I ate or drank that wasn't on my diet.

_____   _____

_____   _____

_____   _____

_____   _____

_____   _____

_____   _____

Remarks: _____

_____

_____

_____

CHEAT SHEET

☐ Good for me! Once again I stayed on my diet!

☐ I cheated. Here is a list of what I ate or drank that wasn't on my diet.

_____	_____
_____	_____
_____	_____
_____	_____
_____	_____

Remarks: _____

_____

_____

_____

CHEAT SHEET

☐ Good for me! Once again I stayed on my diet!

☐ I cheated. Here is a list of what I ate or drank that wasn't on my diet.

_____	_____
_____	_____
_____	_____
_____	_____
_____	_____
_____	_____

Remarks: _____

_____

_____

_____

CHEAT SHEET

☐ Good for me! Once again I stayed on my diet!

☐ I cheated. Here is a list of what I ate or drank that wasn't on my diet.

_____ _____

_____ _____

_____ _____

_____ _____

_____ _____

_____ _____

Remarks: _____

_____

_____

_____

CHEAT SHEET

☐ Good for me! Once again I stayed on my diet!

☐ I cheated. Here is a list of what I ate or drank that wasn't on my diet.

_____ _____

_____ _____

_____ _____

_____ _____

_____ _____

_____ _____

Remarks: _____

_____

_____

_____

CHEAT SHEET

☐ Good for me! Once again I stayed on my diet!

☐ I cheated. Here is a list of what I ate or drank that wasn't on my diet.

_____   _____

_____   _____

_____   _____

_____   _____

_____   _____

_____   _____

Remarks: _____

_____

_____

_____

CHEAT SHEET

☐ Good for me! Once again I stayed on my diet!

☐ I cheated. Here is a list of what I ate or drank that wasn't on my diet.

_____   _____

_____   _____

_____   _____

_____   _____

_____   _____

_____   _____

Remarks: _____

_____

_____

_____

CHEAT SHEET

☐ Good for me! Once again I stayed on my diet!

☐ I cheated. Here is a list of what I ate or drank that wasn't on my diet.

_____   _____

_____   _____

_____   _____

_____   _____

_____   _____

_____

Remarks: _____

_____

_____

_____

CHEAT SHEET

☐ Good for me! Once again I stayed on my diet!

☐ I cheated. Here is a list of what I ate or drank that wasn't on my diet.

_____   _____

_____   _____

_____   _____

_____   _____

_____   _____

_____   _____

Remarks: _____

_____

_____

_____

CHEAT SHEET

☐ Good for me! Once again I stayed on my diet!

☐ I cheated. Here is a list of what I ate or drank that wasn't on my diet.

_____	_____
_____	_____
_____	_____
_____	_____
_____	_____
_____	_____

Remarks: _____

_____

_____

_____

CHEAT SHEET

☐ Good for me! Once again I stayed on my diet!

☐ I cheated. Here is a list of what I ate or drank that wasn't on my diet.

_____   _____

_____   _____

_____   _____

_____   _____

_____   _____

_____   _____

Remarks: _____

_____

_____

_____

CHEAT SHEET

☐ Good for me! Once again I stayed on my diet!

☐ I cheated. Here is a list of what I ate or drank that wasn't on my diet.

_____   _____

_____   _____

_____   _____

_____   _____

_____   _____

_____   _____

Remarks: _____

_____

_____

_____

CHEAT SHEET

☐ Good for me! Once again I stayed on my diet!

☐ I cheated. Here is a list of what I ate or drank that wasn't on my diet.

_____	_____
_____	_____
_____	_____
_____	_____
_____	_____
_____	

Remarks: _____

_____

_____

_____

CHEAT SHEET

☐ Good for me! Once again I stayed on my diet!

☐ I cheated. Here is a list of what I ate or drank that wasn't on my diet.

_____ _____

_____ _____

_____ _____

_____ _____

_____ _____

_____ _____

Remarks: _____

_____

_____

_____

CHEAT SHEET

☐ Good for me! Once again I stayed on my diet!

☐ I cheated. Here is a list of what I ate or drank that wasn't on my diet.

_____   _____

_____   _____

_____   _____

_____   _____

_____   _____

_____   _____

Remarks: _____

_____

_____

_____

CHEAT SHEET

☐ Good for me! Once again I stayed on my diet!

☐ I cheated. Here is a list of what I ate or drank that wasn't on my diet.

_____	_____
_____	_____
_____	_____
_____	_____
_____	_____
_____	_____

Remarks: _____
_____
_____
_____

CHEAT SHEET

☐ Good for me! Once again I stayed on my diet!

☐ I cheated. Here is a list of what I ate or drank that wasn't on my diet.

_____   _____

_____   _____

_____   _____

_____   _____

_____   _____

_____

Remarks: _____

_____

_____

_____

CHEAT SHEET

☐ Good for me! Once again I stayed on my diet!

☐ I cheated. Here is a list of what I ate or drank that wasn't on my diet.

_____   _____

_____   _____

_____   _____

_____   _____

_____   _____

Remarks: _____

_____

_____

_____

CHEAT SHEET

☐ Good for me! Once again I stayed on my diet!

☐ I cheated. Here is a list of what I ate or drank that wasn't on my diet.

_____   _____

_____   _____

_____   _____

_____   _____

_____   _____

_____   _____

Remarks: _____

_____

_____

_____

Date _____

CHEAT SHEET

☐ Good for me! Once again I stayed on my diet!

☐ I cheated. Here is a list of what I ate or drank that wasn't on my diet.

_____   _____

_____   _____

_____   _____

_____   _____

_____   _____

_____

Remarks: _____

_____

_____

_____

CHEAT SHEET

☐ Good for me! Once again I stayed on my diet!

☐ I cheated. Here is a list of what I ate or drank that wasn't on my diet.

_____   _____

_____   _____

_____   _____

_____   _____

_____   _____

_____   _____

Remarks: _____

_____

_____

_____

CHEAT SHEET

☐ Good for me! Once again I stayed on my diet!

☐ I cheated. Here is a list of what I ate or drank that wasn't on my diet.

_____   _____

_____   _____

_____   _____

_____   _____

_____   _____

_____   _____

Remarks: _____

_____

_____

_____

CHEAT SHEET

☐ Good for me! Once again I stayed on my diet!

☐ I cheated. Here is a list of what I ate or drank that wasn't on my diet.

_____   _____

_____   _____

_____   _____

_____   _____

_____   _____

_____   _____

Remarks: _____

_____

_____

_____

CHEAT SHEET

☐ Good for me! Once again I stayed on my diet!

☐ I cheated. Here is a list of what I ate or drank that wasn't on my diet.

_____   _____

_____   _____

_____   _____

_____   _____

_____   _____

Remarks: _____

_____

_____

_____

CHEAT SHEET

☐ Good for me! Once again I stayed on my diet!

☐ I cheated. Here is a list of what I ate or drank that wasn't on my diet.

_____   _____

_____   _____

_____   _____

_____   _____

_____   _____

_____

Remarks: _____

_____

_____

_____

CHEAT SHEET

☐ Good for me! Once again I stayed on my diet!

☐ I cheated. Here is a list of what I ate or drank that wasn't on my diet.

_____   _____

_____   _____

_____   _____

_____   _____

_____   _____

_____   _____

Remarks: _____

_____

_____

_____

CHEAT SHEET

☐ Good for me! Once again I stayed on my diet!

☐ I cheated. Here is a list of what I ate or drank that wasn't on my diet.

_____ _____

_____ _____

_____ _____

_____ _____

_____ _____

_____ _____

Remarks: _____

_____

_____

_____

CHEAT SHEET

☐ Good for me! Once again I stayed on my diet!

☐ I cheated. Here is a list of what I ate or drank that wasn't on my diet.

_____   _____

_____   _____

_____   _____

_____   _____

_____   _____

_____   _____

Remarks: _____

_____

_____

_____

CHEAT SHEET

☐ Good for me! Once again I stayed on my diet!

☐ I cheated. Here is a list of what I ate or drank that wasn't on my diet.

_____   _____

_____   _____

_____   _____

_____   _____

_____   _____

Remarks: _____

_____

_____

_____

CHEAT SHEET

☐ Good for me! Once again I stayed on my diet!

☐ I cheated. Here is a list of what I ate or drank that wasn't on my diet.

_____   _____

_____   _____

_____   _____

_____   _____

_____   _____

Remarks: _____

_____

_____

_____

CHEAT SHEET

☐ Good for me! Once again I stayed on my diet!

☐ I cheated. Here is a list of what I ate or drank that wasn't on my diet.

_____   _____

_____   _____

_____   _____

_____   _____

_____   _____

_____   _____

Remarks: _____

_____

_____

_____

CHEAT SHEET

☐ Good for me! Once again I stayed on my diet!

☐ I cheated. Here is a list of what I ate or drank that wasn't on my diet.

_____	_____
_____	_____
_____	_____
_____	_____
_____	_____
_____	_____

Remarks: _____

_____

_____

_____

CHEAT SHEET

☐ Good for me! Once again I stayed on my diet!

☐ I cheated. Here is a list of what I ate or drank that wasn't on my diet.

_____ _____

_____ _____

_____ _____

_____ _____

_____ _____

_____ _____

Remarks: _____

_____

_____

_____

CHEAT SHEET

☐ Good for me! Once again I stayed on my diet!

☐ I cheated. Here is a list of what I ate or drank that wasn't on my diet.

_____   _____

_____   _____

_____   _____

_____   _____

_____   _____

_____   _____

Remarks: _____

_____

_____

_____

CHEAT SHEET

☐ Good for me! Once again I stayed on my diet!

☐ I cheated. Here is a list of what I ate or drank that wasn't on my diet.

_____   _____
_____   _____
_____   _____
_____   _____
_____   _____
_____   _____

Remarks: _____
_____
_____
_____

CHEAT SHEET

☐ Good for me! Once again I stayed on my diet!

☐ I cheated. Here is a list of what I ate or drank that wasn't on my diet.

_____ _____

_____ _____

_____ _____

_____ _____

_____ _____

Remarks: _____

_____

_____

_____

CHEAT SHEET

☐ Good for me! Once again I stayed on my diet!

☐ I cheated. Here is a list of what I ate or drank that wasn't on my diet.

_____   _____

_____   _____

_____   _____

_____   _____

_____   _____

_____   _____

Remarks: _____

_____

_____

_____

CHEAT SHEET

☐ Good for me! Once again I stayed on my diet!

☐ I cheated. Here is a list of what I ate or drank that wasn't on my diet.

_____	_____
_____	_____
_____	_____
_____	_____
_____	_____
_____	_____

Remarks: _____

_____

_____

_____

CHEAT SHEET

☐ Good for me! Once again I stayed on my diet!

☐ I cheated. Here is a list of what I ate or drank that wasn't on my diet.

_____   _____

_____   _____

_____   _____

_____   _____

_____   _____

_____   _____

Remarks: _____

_____

_____

_____

CHEAT SHEET

☐ Good for me! Once again I stayed on my diet!

☐ I cheated. Here is a list of what I ate or drank that wasn't on my diet.

_____   _____
_____   _____
_____   _____
_____   _____
_____   _____
_____   _____

Remarks: _____
_____
_____
_____

CHEAT SHEET

☐ Good for me! Once again I stayed on my diet!

☐ I cheated. Here is a list of what I ate or drank that wasn't on my diet.

_____   _____

_____   _____

_____   _____

_____   _____

_____   _____

_____   _____

Remarks: _____

_____

_____

_____

CHEAT SHEET

☐ Good for me! Once again I stayed on my diet!

☐ I cheated. Here is a list of what I ate or drank that wasn't on my diet.

_____   _____

_____   _____

_____   _____

_____   _____

_____   _____

Remarks: _____

_____

_____

_____

CHEAT SHEET

☐ Good for me! Once again I stayed on my diet!

☐ I cheated. Here is a list of what I ate or drank that wasn't on my diet.

_____   _____

_____   _____

_____   _____

_____   _____

_____   _____

_____   _____

Remarks: _____

_____

_____

_____

CHEAT SHEET

☐ Good for me! Once again I stayed on my diet!

☐ I cheated. Here is a list of what I ate or drank that wasn't on my diet.

_____	_____
_____	_____
_____	_____
_____	_____
_____	_____
_____	_____

Remarks: _____

_____

_____

_____

CHEAT SHEET

☐ Good for me! Once again I stayed on my diet!

☐ I cheated. Here is a list of what I ate or drank that wasn't on my diet.

_____ _____

_____ _____

_____ _____

_____ _____

_____ _____

_____ _____

Remarks: _____

_____

_____

_____

CHEAT SHEET

☐ Good for me! Once again I stayed on my diet!

☐ I cheated. Here is a list of what I ate or drank that wasn't on my diet.

_____   _____

_____   _____

_____   _____

_____   _____

_____   _____

_____   _____

Remarks: _____

_____

_____

_____

CHEAT SHEET

☐ Good for me! Once again I stayed on my diet!

☐ I cheated. Here is a list of what I ate or drank that wasn't on my diet.

_____   _____

_____   _____

_____   _____

_____   _____

_____   _____

_____   _____

Remarks: _____

_____

_____

_____

CHEAT SHEET

☐ Good for me! Once again I stayed on my diet!

☐ I cheated. Here is a list of what I ate or drank that wasn't on my diet.

_____   _____

_____   _____

_____   _____

_____   _____

_____   _____

_____   _____

Remarks: _____

_____

_____

_____

CHEAT SHEET

☐ Good for me! Once again I stayed on my diet!

☐ I cheated. Here is a list of what I ate or drank that wasn't on my diet.

_____   _____

_____   _____

_____   _____

_____   _____

_____   _____

Remarks: _____

_____

_____

_____

CHEAT SHEET

☐ Good for me! Once again I stayed on my diet!

☐ I cheated. Here is a list of what I ate or drank that wasn't on my diet.

_____   _____

_____   _____

_____   _____

_____   _____

_____   _____

_____   _____

Remarks: _____

_____

_____

_____

CHEAT SHEET

☐ Good for me! Once again I stayed on my diet!

☐ I cheated. Here is a list of what I ate or drank that wasn't on my diet.

_____   _____

_____   _____

_____   _____

_____   _____

_____   _____

_____   _____

Remarks: _____

_____

_____

_____

CHEAT SHEET

☐ Good for me! Once again I stayed on my diet!

☐ I cheated. Here is a list of what I ate or drank that wasn't on my diet.

_____	_____
_____	_____
_____	_____
_____	_____
_____	_____
_____	_____

Remarks: _____

_____

_____

_____

CHEAT SHEET

☐ Good for me! Once again I stayed on my diet!

☐ I cheated. Here is a list of what I ate or drank that wasn't on my diet.

_____   _____

_____   _____

_____   _____

_____   _____

_____   _____

_____   _____

Remarks: _____

_____

_____

_____

CHEAT SHEET

☐ Good for me! Once again I stayed on my diet!

☐ I cheated. Here is a list of what I ate or drank that wasn't on my diet.

_____	_____
_____	_____
_____	_____
_____	_____
_____	_____

Remarks: _____

_____

_____

_____

CHEAT SHEET

☐ Good for me! Once again I stayed on my diet!

☐ I cheated. Here is a list of what I ate or drank that wasn't on my diet.

_____   _____

_____   _____

_____   _____

_____   _____

_____   _____

_____   _____

Remarks: _____

_____

_____

_____

CHEAT SHEET

☐ Good for me! Once again I stayed on my diet!

☐ I cheated. Here is a list of what I ate or drank that wasn't on my diet.

_____	_____
_____	_____
_____	_____
_____	_____
_____	_____
_____	_____

Remarks: _____

_____

_____

_____

CHEAT SHEET

☐ Good for me! Once again I stayed on my diet!

☐ I cheated. Here is a list of what I ate or drank that wasn't on my diet.

_____ _____

_____ _____

_____ _____

_____ _____

_____ _____

_____ _____

Remarks: _____

_____

_____

_____